HOW DOES THE ANTI-INFLAMMATORY DIET WORK?

Gary S. Rains

Contents

Chapter One

Muffins With Spinach

MAKES 12 MUFFINS / TIME TO PREPARE: 15 MINUTES / TIME TO COOK: 15 MINUTES

• THE MEDIEVAL

Muffins with spinach? Why not include spinach alongside zucchini, carrots, pumpkin, and beets in baked goods? These muffins are a hit with kids, yet they have no idea they include vegetables. For good luck, tell them they're green.

Spray for cooking

2 cups spinach, packed

two eggs

14 cup honey (raw)

extra-virgin olive oil, 3 teaspoons

1 teaspoon essence of vanilla

1 cup flour made from oats

1 tablespoon almond flour

2 tblsp. baking powder

1 teaspoon bicarbonate of soda

12 teaspoon sodium chloride

1 tsp. black pepper, freshly ground

1. Preheat the oven to 350 degrees Fahrenheit.

2. Spray 12 muffin cups with cooking spray or line them with paper liners.

3. Combine the spinach, eggs, honey, olive oil, and vanilla in a food processor. Blend until completely smooth.

4. Combine the oat flour, almond flour, baking powder, baking soda, salt, and pepper in a medium mixing basin. Mix the spinach mixture thoroughly in the bowl.

5. Fill each muffin cup halfway with batter. Place the muffins in the preheated oven for about 15 minutes, or until lightly browned and firm to the touch in the centre.

6. Place the pan on a cooling rack and let aside for 10 minutes before removing the muffins.

VEGAN TIP: For each egg, replace it with a mixture of 1 tablespoon powdered flaxseed and 3 tablespoons water.

PALEO TIP: Instead of combining almond and oat flours, use solely almond flour.

EACH SERVING

108 calories; 6 grammes of total fat

12 g total carbohydrates

6 g sugar; 1 g fibre

3g protein; 217mg sodium

Chapter Two

Herb Scramble with Cherry Tomatoes Sauté

PREP TIME: 5 MINUTES / COOK TIME: 10 MINUTES / SERVES 2

- PALEO Diet
- THE MEDIEVAL
- SAVING TIME

In this high-protein breakfast, oregano, garlic, and tomatoes are classic Mediterranean flavours. Avocado slices include vitamins as well as beneficial fats. This is the ideal breakfast to get you ready for the day ahead.

four eggs

2 teaspoons fresh oregano, chopped

1 tablespoon olive oil (extra virgin)

1 cup halved cherry tomatoes

12 chopped garlic cloves

12 sliced avocado

1. Whisk the eggs and oregano together in a medium mixing basin until thoroughly blended.

2. In a large skillet, heat the oil over medium heat. Add the olive oil once the pan is heated.

3. Pour the eggs into the skillet and scramble them using a heat-resistant spatula or a wooden spoon. Place the eggs on a serving platter.

4. Add the garlic and cherry tomatoes to the pan and cook for about 2 minutes. Place the tomatoes on top of the eggs and garnish with avocado slices.

Alert for Sensitivity

EACH SERVING

310 calories; 26 grammes of total fat

10g total carbohydrates

3 g sugar; 5 g fibre

13g protein; 131mg sodium

Chapter Three

"Frittata" of mushrooms

PREP TIME: 15 MINUTES / COOK TIME: 20 MINUTES / SERVES 6

• VEGETARIAN

This frittata isn't actually a frittata at all; instead of eggs, a tasty protein basis is provided by a garbanzo bean batter. For breakfast, serve with fresh fruit, and for lunch or dinner, serve with a simple green salad.

a total of 112 cup chickpea flour

12 quarts water

1 tblsp. salt

2 tbsp olive oil extra-virgin

1 tiny chopped red onion

2 pints mushrooms, sliced

1 teaspoon turmeric powder

12 teaspoon cumin powder

1 tblsp. salt

12 teaspoon black pepper, freshly ground

2 tablespoons fresh parsley, chopped

1. Preheat the oven to 350 degrees Fahrenheit.

2. Slowly whisk the water into the chickpea flour in a small bowl; season with salt and leave aside.

3. Heat the olive oil in a big cast iron or oven-safe skillet over high heat. Add the onion after the oil is heated. Cook for 3 to 5 minutes, or until onion is cooked and transparent. Add the mushrooms and cook for another 5 minutes. Sauté for 1 minute with the turmeric, cumin, salt, and pepper.

4. Drizzle the batter over the vegetables and top with parsley. Preheat the oven to 350°F and roast the skillet for 20 to 25 minutes.

5. Serve at room temperature or heated.

PALEO TIP: Skip the chickpea batter if you're following the Paleo Action Plan. 6 eggs, beaten until frothy Pour the eggs over the vegetables that have been sautéed.

MEDITERRANEAN TIP: Crumble 2 ounces of goat's milk feta cheese over the batter before baking if you're following the Mediterranean Action Plan.

TIP: Buy the red onions already chopped and the mushrooms already sliced to save time.

ACTION PLAN TIP: If you're following the Vegan or Mediterranean Action Plans, double the recipe to ensure you have enough leftovers for the rest of the week.

EACH SERVING

240 calories; 8 grammes of total fat

34g total carbohydrates

7g sugar; 10g fibre

11g protein; 792mg sodium

Chapter Four

Lettuce Wraps with Cucumber and Smoked Salmon

PREP TIME: 10 MINUTES / SERVES 4

• PALEO Diet

• SAVING TIME

Any breakfast or lunch table will benefit from the addition of these wraps. Salmon is abundant in omega-3 fatty acids and is a quick and easy high-protein substitute for eggs. Because they have fewer seeds, English cucumbers, also known as seedless cucumbers, are easier to digest and have a sweeter flavour.

8 butter lettuce leaves, large

12 English cucumbers, thinly sliced

smoked salmon, 8 ounces, divided

1 tablespoon fresh chives, chopped

4 tablespoons Almost Caesar Salad Dressing (recipe here)

1. Arrange the lettuce leaves in a single layer on a serving dish.

2. Arrange the cucumber slices evenly among the lettuce leaves. 2 ounces smoked salmon on top of each leaf

3. Sprinkle with chives and spread 1 spoonful of Almost Caesar Salad Dressing over each wrap.

MEDITERRANEAN TIP: For each wrap, add 2 tablespoons goat cheese.

EACH SERVING

107 calories; 5 grammes of total fat

6 g total carbohydrates

4 g sugar; 1 g fibre

11g protein; 1261mg sodium

Chapter Five

Hash of Sweet Potatoes

PREP TIME: 15 MINUTES / COOK TIME: 15 MINUTES / SERVES 4

• VEGETARIAN

• PALEO Diet

• THE MEDIEVAL

Sweet potatoes, mushrooms, and greens combine to provide a delicious and nutritious lunch. Purchase pre-sliced onions and mushrooms to save time, or prepare a double batch on the weekend to enjoy during the week.

coconut oil, 2 tablespoons

12 onion, thinly sliced

1 cup mushrooms, sliced

1 thinly chopped garlic clove

2 big cooked sweet potatoes, cut into 12-inch cubes

1 cup Swiss chard, finely chopped

12 CUP VEGAN BROTH

1 tblsp. salt

14 teaspoon pepper, freshly ground

1 tablespoon fresh thyme, chopped

1 tablespoon fresh sage, chopped

1. Melt the coconut oil in a large skillet over high heat.

2. Stir in the garlic, onion, and mushrooms. Cook for 8 minutes, or until the onions and mushrooms are soft.

3. Combine the sweet potatoes, Swiss chard, and vegetable broth in a large mixing bowl. 5 minutes of cooking

4. Add the salt, pepper, thyme, and sage and mix well.

Vegans can enhance their protein intake by adding 1 cup of cooked black beans. Crumble Easy Turkey Breakfast Sausage (recipe here) into the hash if you're following the Mediterranean or Paleo diets.

ACTION PLAN TIP: If you're following the Vegan, Paleo, or Time-Saving Action Plans, double the recipe to ensure you have enough leftovers for the rest of the week.

EACH SERVING

212 calories; 7 grammes of total fat

35g total carbohydrates

2 g sugar; 6 g fibre

30g protein; 708mg sodium

4 SERVINGS CUCUMBERS-YOGURT DIP / PREP TIME: 15 MINUTES

- VEGETARIAN
- PALEO Diet
- THE MEDIEVAL
- SAVING TIME

This is a traditional tzatziki sauce made using coconut yoghurt instead of dairy yoghurt. You can also use plain, unsweetened almond milk yoghurt. Enable the dip to sit for at least one hour before serving to allow the flavours to meld. Use as a sauce with chicken or fish, or serve with fresh vegetables or gluten-free crackers.

1 peeled and shredded cucumber

1 cup coconut yoghurt, plain

1 minced garlic clove

1 sliced scallion

2 tablespoons fresh dill, chopped

1 tblsp. salt

2 tbsp lemon juice, freshly squeezed

2 tbsp olive oil extra-virgin

1. Drain the cucumber shredded in a fine-mesh sieve.

2. Combine the yoghurt, garlic, scallion, dill, salt, and lemon juice in a small bowl.

3. Stir in the cucumber and transfer to a serving bowl.

4. Drizzle with olive oil just before serving.

EACH SERVING

104 calories; 9 grammes of total fat

7g total carbohydrates

2 g sugar; 3 g fibre

1 gramme protein; 636 milligrammes sodium

Chapter Six

Dip with white beans

PREP TIME: 15 MINUTES / SERVES 4–6 PEOPLE

• VEGETARIAN

• THE MEDIEVAL

• SAVING TIME

Simple, quick, and delectable. What's not to like about that? To make it more hummus-like, replace the white beans with garbanzo beans.

1 can (15 oz.) white beans, rinsed and drained

1 clove garlic

1 tablespoon almond butter or tahini

extra-virgin olive oil, 3 teaspoons

14 cup pitted green olives, diced

1 tablespoon parsley, chopped

14 teaspoon kosher salt

2 tbsp lemon juice, freshly squeezed

1. Combine the white beans, garlic, and tahini in a food processor. Slowly drizzle in the olive oil in a thin, steady stream while the machine is on low. Thin the dip with some water if it's too thick.

2. Combine the olives, parsley, and salt in a bowl. To blend, pulse. Add the lemon juice and mix well.

3. Serve with raw vegetables and gluten-free crackers in a serving bowl.

Alert for Sensitivity

EACH SERVING

239 calories; 14 grammes of total fat

25g total carbohydrates

0g sugar; 6g fibre

9g protein; 358mg sodium

Chapter Seven

Jicama Slices with Mashed Avocado

PREP TIME: 15 MINUTES / SERVES 4

- VEGETARIAN
- PALEO Diet
- THE MEDIEVAL
- SAVING TIME

Avocado can be incorporated into almost any diet. This version of guacamole combines creamy, nutrient-dense avocado with turmeric, an anti-inflammatory spice native to southwest India. Jicama is high in fibre and stimulates the growth of "good" bacteria in the gut, so consume it guilt-free.

2 pitted ripe avocados

1 chopped scallion

2 tablespoons fresh cilantro, chopped

12 teaspoon turmeric powder

12 lemon juice

1 tblsp. salt

14 teaspoon black pepper, freshly ground

1 peeled jicama, cut into 14-inch thick slices

1. Combine the avocado, scallion, cilantro, turmeric, lemon juice, salt, and pepper in a small bowl. Mix the ingredients together until they're well combined but still chunky.

2. Garnish with jicama slices.

INGREDIENT HINT: Avocado quickly browns. Place plastic wrap on on top of the dip, smoothing it down so there are no air pockets, to slow the oxidation process.

EACH SERVING

270 calories; 20 grammes of total fat

24g total carbohydrates

4 g sugar; 15 g fibre

3g protein; 595mg sodium

Chapter Eight

Broccoli Dip with Cream

PREP TIME: 20 MINUTES / COOK TIME: 5 MINUTES / MAKES ABOUT 2 CUPS

- VEGETARIAN
- PALEO Diet
- THE MEDIEVAL

When broccoli is combined with garlic, avocado, and green onions, it takes on a sweet, nutty flavour. Dollop it on omelettes or grilled meats in addition to using it as a dip for snacks like Sweet Potato Chips (see here). It transforms an ordinary day into something extraordinary.

broccoli florets, 1 cup

1 clove garlic

1 roughly chopped scallion

34 cup plain unsweetened almond or coconut yoghurt

12 avocadoes

1 tablespoon lemon juice, freshly squeezed

1 tblsp. salt

12 teaspoon dill, dry

1 teaspoon red pepper flakes

1. Place a steamer basket in a medium saucepan with 2 inches of water and place it over medium-high heat.

2. Add the broccoli to the steamer basket, cover, and steam for 5 minutes, or until the broccoli turns brilliant green. Drain the broccoli and remove the pan from the heat.

3. Combine the garlic, scallion, yoghurt, avocado, lemon juice, salt, dill, and red pepper flakes in a food processor. Pulse the mixture a few times until it looks coarsely chopped.

4. Add the broccoli and process until fully blended; the mixture should be chunky and not completely smooth. Serve with Sweet Potato Chips (recipe here) or fresh vegetable sticks like as carrots and celery.

TIP: Store this dip in an airtight jar in the refrigerator for up to one week.

14 CUP PER SERVING

82 calories; 7 grammes of total fat

7g total carbohydrates

1 g sugar; 4 g fibre

1 gramme protein; 628 milligrammes sodium

Chapter Nine

Wraps with smoked trout and mango

PREP TIME: 15 MINUTES / SERVES 4

• PALEO Diet

• THE MEDIEVAL

• SAVING TIME

The sweetness of the mango complements the delicate, smoky flavour of smoked fish. Instead of using the lettuce leaves as a wrap, shred them and use them to make a salad.

4 huge leaves of green lettuce, thick stalks removed

4 oz. smoked trout (distributed)

1 cup mango chunks, split

1 sliced and split scallion

2 tablespoons lemon juice (distributed)

1. Lay the lettuce leaves out flat on a table. Top each leaf with equal amounts of fish and mango. Scatter the scallions over top and drizzle with lemon juice.

2. Burrito-style wrap the lettuce leaves and arrange them seam-side down on a serving platter.

VEGAN TIP: For a smokey flavour, replace the smoked fish with 1 cup cooked black beans combined with 12 teaspoon chipotle powder.

EACH SERVING

Calories: 108; Total Fat: 3g;

13g total carbohydrates

10 g sugar; 3 g fibre

9g protein; 52mg sodium

SERVES 4 / TIME TO PREPARE: 20 MINUTES / TIME TO COOK: 20 MINUTES

• VEGETARIAN

• PALEO Diet

• THE MEDIEVAL

Although kale chips are widely accessible and simple to prepare, making your own ensures that you know precisely what's in them and that you get all of the anti-inflammatory benefits. They must be consumed within 24 hours otherwise the crunch will be lost.

1 kale bunch, washed and dried completely, ribs removed, and cut into 2-inch strips

2 tbsp olive oil extra-virgin

1 tablespoon salt

1. Preheat the oven to 275 degrees Fahrenheit.

2. In a large mixing basin, toss the kale with the olive oil with your hands until the kale is equally covered.

3. Place the kale on a baking sheet and spread it out in a single layer. Season with salt and pepper.

4. Bake for about 20 minutes, or until the kale is crisp, on a prepared baking sheet. Halfway through the baking time, flip the chips over to crisp the other side.

5. Before serving, allow the chips to cool slightly.

TIP: Keep the cooled chips at room temperature in an airtight container.

EACH SERVING

93 calories; 7 grammes of total fat

7g total carbohydrates

0g sugar; 1g fibre

2g protein; 497mg sodium

Chapter Ten

Zucchini Sticks with Smoked Turkey Wrapping

PREP TIME: 10 MINUTES / SERVES 4

- PALEO Diet
- THE MEDIEVAL
- SAVING TIME

This late-afternoon—or anytime—snack features moderate smokiness from the turkey, peppery arugula, and the pleasant crunch of a zucchini stick. These are great for taking to work or on a picnic. Protein will keep you fuller for longer than anything from a vending machine.

8 thin smoked turkey slices

2 zucchini, lengthwise quartered

1 cup arugula leaves, divided

1 tsp salt

1. On a work surface, place 1 slice of smoked turkey. 1 zucchini stick, 14 cup arugula, and a pinch of salt on top

2. Wrap the turkey around the vegetables and place seam-side down on a plate. Rep with the rest of the ingredients.

3. Refrigerate until ready to serve.

COOKING TIP: Drizzle with a little olive oil and lemon juice for a taste boost.

EACH SERVING

137 calories; 3 grammes of total fat

6 g total carbohydrates

2 g sugar; 1 g fibre

21g protein; 1450mg sodium

Chapter Eleven

Chickpeas with a Crunch and a Kick

PREP TIME: 10 MINUTES / COOK TIME: 30 TO 40 MINUTES / MAKES 1 CUP

• VEGETARIAN

• THE MEDIEVAL

A filling snack that's simple to store and have on hand for a quick boost. It's better to consume these within five days of purchase because they lose their crunch after that time. It's less expensive to make them yourself than to buy them, plus you'll know precisely what's in them.

1 drained 15-ounce can chickpeas

1 tblsp. salt

12 teaspoon cumin powder

12 teaspoon powdered onion

12 teaspoon turmeric powder

12 teaspoon powdered chipotle

a quarter teaspoon of garlic powder

2 tbsp olive oil extra-virgin

1. Preheat the oven to 375 degrees Fahrenheit.

2. Using a paper towel, dry the drained chickpeas.

3. Combine the salt, cumin, onion powder, turmeric, chipotle powder, and garlic powder in a small bowl.

4. Combine the dry chickpeas and olive oil in a medium mixing dish. Stir the chickpeas gently to coat them in the oil.

5. Drizzle the chickpeas with the salt mixture. Stir until everything is evenly covered.

6. Spread the chickpeas in a single layer on a wide baking sheet with raised sides (to avoid them from rolling off). Bake for 30 to 40 minutes, stirring regularly, or until the chickpeas are dry and crunchy on the baking sheet.

7. Allow to cool completely before consuming.

TIP: If you're not going to consume them right away, keep them in an airtight jar at room temperature.

TIP: Before baking the chickpeas, line the baking sheet with parchment paper to save time. Cleaning up will be a breeze.

TIP: If you're following the Vegan or Mediterranean Action Plans, double the recipe to ensure you have enough leftovers for the rest of the week.

14 CUP PER SERVING

192 calories; 10 grammes of total fat

18g total carbohydrates

1 g sugar; 5 g fibre

8g protein; 593mg sodium

Chapter Twelve

Chips of Sweet Potato

PREP TIME: 20 MINUTES / COOK TIME: 2 HOURS / SERVES 4 TO 6

• VEGETARIAN

• PALEO Diet

• THE MEDIEVAL

Sweet potato chips are incredibly excellent, either alone or with Creamy Broccoli Dip (see here) (see here). Slice the sweet potatoes as thinly as possible for a crispy chip. Use a mandoline or the food processor's thin-slicing disc. You're still in luck if all you have is a sharp knife and patience. Thicker chips are chewier than crispy chips, but they're just as tasty.

2 big sweet potatoes, thinly sliced

extra-virgin olive oil, 3 teaspoons

1 tablespoon salt

1. Preheat the oven to 250 degrees Fahrenheit.

2. Place the oven rack in the middle of the oven.

3. Toss the sweet potato pieces with the olive oil in a large mixing dish. Arrange the slices on two baking pans in a single layer. Season with salt and pepper.

4. Bake the sheets for around 2 hours in a preheated oven, rotating the pans and flipping the chips after 1 hour.

5. Remove the chips from the oven when they are gently browned and crisp. Some may be a little squishy at first, but as they cool, they will crisp up. Allow 10 minutes for the chips to cool before serving.

6. Serve right away. Within a few hours, the chips have lost their crunch.

EACH SERVING

267 calories; 11 grammes of total fat

42g total carbohydrates

1 g sugar; 6 g fibre

2g protein; 482mg sodium

Chapter Thirteen

Mini Muffins for Snacks

PREP TIME: 20 MINUTES / COOK TIME: 15 TO 20 MINUTES

MAKES 24

• THE MEDIEVAL

Defend yourself from a snack attack with these muffins, which have no added sugar and are excellent for any time of day. Make ahead of time to have on hand, or double the recipe and freeze. Warm with a sprinkling of raw honey, they're delicious.

14 cup ultra-virgin olive oil + a little extra for frying

1 tablespoon almond flour

1 cup rice flour (brown)

1 tablespoon powdered sugar

12 teaspoon sodium chloride

1 teaspoon cinnamon powder

four eggs

1 carrot, shredded

1 cup pumpkin puree

1. Preheat the oven to 375 degrees Fahrenheit.

2. Use cupcake liners or brush a mini-muffin tin with olive oil to line it.

3. Combine the almond flour, brown rice flour, baking powder, salt, and cinnamon in a medium mixing basin.

4. Combine the eggs, carrots, pumpkin, and olive oil in a mixing bowl. Stir until everything is completely blended.

5. Scoop about three-quarters of the batter into each muffin cup.

6. Bake the muffins for 15 minutes in a preheated oven, or until they are gently browned. Remove the muffins from the tin and cool for 10 minutes before removing them.

If you're following the Vegan Action Plan, substitute 4 tablespoons ground flaxseed with 8 ounces water in place of the eggs.

Replace the brown rice flour with coconut flour if you're following the Paleo Action Plan.

EACH SERVING (1 muffin)

65 calories; 4 g total fat

7g total carbohydrates

1 g sugar; 1 g fibre

2g protein; 66mg sodium

Chapter Fourteen

Chia-Strawberry Ice Pops

MAKES 6 ICE POPS / TIME TO PREPARE: 20 MINUTES / TIME TO FREEZE: 5 HOURS

- VEGETARIAN
- PALEO Diet
- THE MEDIEVAL

These ice pops are light and refreshing, and you can create them with whatever frozen or fresh fruit you prefer. When using fresh fruit, mash it first before mixing it with the rest of the ingredients. You'll avoid biting into overly huge frozen fruit bits this way.

2 cup thawed frozen unsweetened strawberries

1 tablespoon lemon juice, freshly squeezed

1 coconut milk (15-ounce) can

chia seeds, 1 tbsp

1 teaspoon essence of vanilla

1. Follow the manufacturer's directions to make six ice pop moulds.

2. Combine the strawberries, lemon juice, coconut milk, chia seeds, and vanilla in a medium mixing dish. Allow 5 minutes for the chia seeds to thicken slightly before serving. This makes filling the moulds much easier.

3. Divide the mixture evenly between the moulds. In each mould, place one ice pop stick. Freeze the pops for 5 hours or overnight until they are solid.

Use muffin tins instead of ice pop moulds if you don't have any. Before filling the tins, line them with parchment paper. Because it's difficult to keep sticks erect in the unfrozen mixture, freeze them for 2 hours before inserting them.

EACH SERVING (1 ice pop)

187 calories; 17 grammes of total fat

9g total carbohydrates

6 g sugar; 3 g fibre

2g protein; 11mg sodium

Chapter Fifteen

Soup with Roasted Vegetables

6–8 SERVINGS / TIME TO PREPARE: 30 MINUTES / TIME TO COOK: 40 MINUTES

- VEGETARIAN
- PALEO Diet
- THE MEDIEVAL

This recipe is versatile, bright, and tasty, and it can be made with any vegetables you have on hand. This is a great way to use up leftover roasted vegetables or anything else in the fridge that's about to go bad. Roasting brings out the sweetness and depth of flavour. This soup appeals to even the pickiest vegetable eaters.

4 carrots, cut in half lengthwise

12 florets from a head of cauliflower

2 cups butternut squash, diced

3 shallots, lengthwise halved

3 quartered Roma tomatoes

4 cloves garlic

12 cup olive oil (extra virgin)

1 tblsp. salt

14 teaspoon black pepper, freshly ground

4–6 cups veggie broth or water

1. Preheat the oven to 400 degrees Fahrenheit.

2. Combine the carrots, cauliflower, butternut squash, shallots, tomatoes, and garlic in a large mixing basin. Toss the vegetables in the olive oil, salt, and pepper to coat.

3. Arrange the vegetables in a single layer on a rimmed baking sheet. Place the sheet in the oven and roast for about 25 minutes, or until the vegetables begin to brown.

4. Place the roasted veggies in a large Dutch oven and cook on high. Bring to a boil with enough water to cover the vegetables. Reduce the heat to a low heat and continue to cook the soup for another 10 minutes.

5. Pour the soup into a blender and puree until smooth, working in batches if necessary.

Alert for Sensitivity

COOKING TIP: Purée the soup with 12 cup coconut milk for a creamy soup.

TIP FOR SAVING TIME: If you're following the Vegan or Paleo Action Plan, double the recipe to ensure you have enough for leftovers later in the week.

EACH SERVING

197 calories; 17 grammes of total fat

13g total carbohydrates

5 g sugar; 3 g fibre

2g protein; 426mg sodium

Chapter Sixteen

Broth with Mushrooms

PREP TIME: 15 MINUTES / COOK TIME: 10 MINUTES / SERVES 4

• VEGETARIAN

• PALEO Diet

• THE MEDIEVAL

A small lunch or snack with this relaxing soup. Mushrooms contain anti-inflammatory properties and help to strengthen our immune systems. Buy pre-sliced onions and mushrooms, as well as pre-chopped celery, to save time in the kitchen.

1 tablespoon olive oil (extra virgin)

1 onion, halved and thinly sliced

3 thinly chopped garlic cloves

1 finely sliced celery stalk

1 pound thinly sliced mushrooms

1 tblsp. salt

12 teaspoon black pepper, freshly ground

1 tsp. nutmeg

4 c. vegetable stock

2 tablespoons fresh tarragon, chopped

1. Heat the olive oil in a big pot over high heat.
2. Add the celery, onion, and garlic. 3 minutes of sautéing
3. Season with salt, pepper, and nutmeg. Cook for another 5 to 10 minutes.
4. Bring the soup to a boil with the veggie broth. Reduce the heat to a low setting. Cook for a further 5 minutes.
5. Finish by adding the tarragon and serving.

PALEO & MEDITERRANEAN TIP: For a heartier soup, use chicken stock instead of vegetable broth and add 1 cup cooked chicken or fish if following the Mediterranean or Paleo Action Plan.

EACH SERVING

111 calories; 5 grammes of total fat

9g total carbohydrates

4 g sugar; 2 g fibre

9g protein; 1357mg sodium

Chapter Seventeen

Soup with fried sage and pumpkin

PREP TIME: 15 MINUTES / COOK TIME: 10 MINUTES / SERVES 4

- VEGETARIAN
- PALEO Diet
- THE MEDIEVAL

Pumpkin is no longer just for Thanksgiving. Because this soup is made with canned pumpkin, you can eat it whenever the mood strikes. You might be tempted to forgo the fried sage, but sage has anti-inflammatory and antioxidant effects, and it pairs beautifully with the earthiness of the pumpkin.

4 tbsp olive oil (extra virgin)

1 chopped onion

2 garlic cloves, cut into thick slices of 18 inches

1 pumpkin purée (15 ounces)

4 c. vegetable stock

chipotle powder, 2 tablespoons

1 tblsp. salt

12 teaspoon black pepper, freshly ground

12 cup oil (vegetable)

12 stemmed sage leaves

1. Heat the olive oil, onion, and garlic in a big, heavy Dutch over high heat. Cook for 5 minutes, or until the vegetables are starting to brown.

2. Combine the pumpkin, vegetable broth, chipotle powder, salt, and pepper in a large mixing bowl. Bring the water to a boil. Reduce the heat to low and continue to cook for another 5 minutes.

3. Heat a medium sauté pan over high heat while the soup is boiling. Heat the vegetable oil until it is hot.

4. Carefully place each sage leaf in the oil and fry for 1 minute, or until crisp. Transfer the sage to paper towels to drain using a slotted spoon. Remove the vegetable oil once it has cooled.

5. Ladle the soup into bowls (purée the soup first if desired), and top with 3 fried sage leaves each dish.

INGREDIENT TIP: You can cook the sage leaves in extra-virgin olive oil, but because the oil is dumped afterward, it's better to use a less-expensive oil. Make sage leaves as soon as possible because they only stay crisp for a few hours.

ACTION PLAN TIP: If you're following the Paleo Action Plan, double the recipe to ensure you have enough leftovers for the rest of the week.

EACH SERVING

379 calories; 20 grammes of total fat

45g total carbohydrates

17g sugar; 18g fibre

10g protein; 1365mg sodium

Chapter Eighteen

Soup with Lentils and Carrots with Ginger

PREP TIME: 15 MINUTES / COOK TIME: 10 MINUTES / SERVES 4 TO 6

- VEGETARIAN
- THE MEDIEVAL

Protein, iron, and fibre are abundant in lentils. They go well with ginger, which helps digestion and lowers inflammation. Before serving, top the soup with crumbled goat cheese if you're following the Mediterranean Action Plan.

coconut oil, 1 tablespoon

2 thinly sliced carrots

1 peeled and thinly sliced small white onion

2 peeled and thinly sliced garlic cloves

1 tablespoon fresh ginger, chopped

3 cups veggie broth or water

1 (15-ounce) can drained and washed lentils

2 tablespoons fresh cilantro or parsley, chopped

1 tblsp. salt

14 teaspoon black pepper, freshly ground

1. Melt the coconut oil in a large pot over medium-high heat. Carrots, onion, garlic, and ginger should be added now. 5 minutes of sautéing

2. Fill the saucepan halfway with water and come to a boil. Reduce the heat to low and cook the carrots for about 5 minutes, or until they are soft.

3. Combine the lentils, cilantro, salt, and pepper in a mixing bowl. Serve with a good stir.

TIP: If you're following the Vegan or Mediterranean Action Plans, double the recipe to ensure you have enough leftovers for the rest of the week.

EACH SERVING

207 calories; 5 grammes of total fat

28g total carbohydrates

5 g sugar; 10 g fibre

14g protein; 1430mg sodium

Chapter Nineteen

Soup with Squash and Coconut Curry

4–6 SERVINGS / 15 MINUTE PREP TIME / 4 HOUR COOK TIME

• VEGETARIAN

• PALEO Diet

• THE MEDIEVAL

• SAVING TIME

This soup is made in a slow cooker: simply add the ingredients in the morning and return home to a scented home and a ready-to-eat meal. Garnish with shredded coconut, chopped cashews, and sliced green apple to make the soup more appealing.

coconut oil, 2 tablespoons

1 pound peeled and cut into 1-inch cubes butternut squash

1 cauliflower head, sliced into 1-inch pieces

ı sliced onion

curry powder (1 tablespoon)

12 cup apple juice (no sugar added)

4 c. vegetable stock

1 coconut milk can (13.5 oz.)

1 tblsp. salt

14 teaspoon white pepper, freshly ground

14 cup cilantro, chopped, divided

1. Toss together the butternut squash, cauliflower, onion, curry powder, apple juice, vegetable broth, coconut milk, salt, and white pepper in a slow cooker. Set the timer for 4 hours on high.

2. Serve the soup as is or puree it until smooth before serving.

3. Add the cilantro as a garnish.

ACTION PLAN TIP: If you're following the Vegan, Paleo, or Time-Saving Action Plans, double the recipe to ensure you have extra leftovers for the following week.

EACH SERVING

416 calories; 31 grammes of total fat

30g total carbohydrates

13 g sugar; 7 g fibre

10g protein; 1387mg sodium

Chapter Twenty

Soup with Soba Noodles and Spinach

PREP TIME: 15 MINUTES / COOK TIME: 10 MINUTES / SERVES 4

• VEGETARIAN

• THE MEDIEVAL

Look for 100% buckwheat soba noodles, as gluten-containing soba noodles are not anti-inflammatory. Buckwheat soba noodles are quick to cook and delicious hot or cold. If shiitake mushrooms are unavailable or too expensive, use another type of mushroom.

coconut oil, 2 tablespoons

8 oz. stemmed and thinly sliced shiitake mushrooms

4 thinly sliced scallions

1 minced garlic clove

1 tablespoon fresh ginger, minced

1 tblsp. salt

4 c. vegetable stock

3 quarts of water

buckwheat soba noodles, 4 oz

1 bunch washed and cut into strips spinach

1 tablespoon lemon juice, freshly squeezed

1. Melt the coconut oil in a large pot over medium heat.
2. Combine the mushrooms, scallions, garlic, ginger, and salt in a mixing bowl. 5 minutes of sautéing
3. Bring the vegetable broth and water to a boil in the pot. Cook for 5 minutes after adding the soba noodles.
4. Turn off the heat in the pot. Combine the spinach and lemon juice in a mixing bowl. Serve immediately.

ACTION PLAN TIP: If you're following the Vegan or Mediterranean Action Plans, double the recipe to ensure you have enough leftovers for the rest of the week.

EACH SERVING

255 calories; 9 grammes of total fat

34g total carbohydrates

4 g sugar; 4 g fibre

13g protein; 1774mg sodium

Chapter Twenty-one

Soup with Sweet Potatoes and Rice

4–6 SERVINGS / 15 MINUTES TO PREPARE / 15 MINUTES TO COOK

• VEGETARIAN

Because it's fantastic to make with leftover rice and vegetables, this easy and comforting soup may be termed "leftover soup." The soup has a moderate flavour; add red pepper flakes or a teaspoon or two of coconut aminos to heat it up.

4 c. vegetable stock

1 large peeled sweet potato, cut into 1-inch cubes

2 coarsely chopped onions

2 thinly chopped garlic cloves

2 teaspoons fresh ginger, minced

1 broccolini bunch, cut into 1-inch chunks

1 cup basmati rice, cooked

14 cup cilantro leaves, fresh

1. Bring the broth to a boil in a large Dutch oven over high heat.
2. Combine the sweet potato, onion, garlic, and ginger in a mixing bowl. Cook for 5 to 8 minutes, or until the sweet potato is tender.
3. Add the broccolini and continue to cook for another 3 minutes.
4. Turn off the heat in the pan. Combine the rice and cilantro in a mixing bowl.

MEDITERRANEAN& PALEO TIP: Instead of vegetable broth, use chicken broth if following the Mediterranean or Paleo Action Plans. If you're following the Paleo Action Plan, you can also skip the rice.

EACH SERVING

167 calories; 2 grammes of total fat

29g total carbohydrates

7 g sugar; 3 g fibre

8g protein; 789mg sodium

Chapter Twenty-two

Stew with Broccoli and Lentils

PREP TIME: 15 MINUTES / COOK TIME: 30 MINUTES / SERVES 4

• VEGETARIAN

• THE MEDIEVAL

The Mediterranean tastes of this stew come from green olives and Italian parsley. Broccoli and lentils are high in fibre, making this stew filling. On a cold day, this is a fantastic supper to warm you up.

1 tablespoon extra-virgin olive oil, with a little extra to drizzle

1 finely chopped tiny onion

1 sliced tiny carrot

2 garlic cloves, minced

2 c. vegetable stock

1 cup green or brown lentils, dry

1 teaspoon oregano, dry

broccoli florets, 6 cups

1 tblsp. salt

14 teaspoon black pepper, freshly ground

12 cup pitted green olives, sliced

14 cup fresh Italian parsley, chopped

1. Heat the olive oil in a big pot over high heat.

2. Combine the onion, carrot, and garlic in a bowl. 5 minutes of sautéing

3. Bring to a boil the vegetable broth, lentils, and oregano. Reduce the heat to a low setting. Cook the lentils in the soup for 15 to 20 minutes, or until they are soft.

4. Add the broccoli, cover, and cook for another 5 minutes.

5. Turn off the heat and add the olives and parsley to the saucepan. Stir in some water if the soup is too thick.

6. Ladle the soup into bowls and sprinkle with olive oil before serving.

EACH SERVING

182 calories; 6 g total fat

24g total carbohydrates

5 g sugar; 9 g fibre

11g protein; 1233mg sodium

Chapter Twenty-three

Kasha and Winter Squash Stew

4 SERVINGS / 15 MINUTE PREP TIME / 4 HOUR COOK TIME

• VEGETARIAN

• THE MEDIEVAL

• SAVING TIME

Buckwheat is toasted in Kasha. It's not a grain, but rather a grass. It's meaty and rich, and goes well with winter squash. To retain the texture and nutrition of the kale, it is added at the end of the cooking period. It loses more nutrients when it cooks, as it does with other greens. This soup will provide you with both comfort and nourishment.

1 tablespoon olive oil (extra virgin)

2 pounds peeled and diced winter squash

1 thinly sliced fennel bulb

2 leeks, thinly cut white part only

2 chopped garlic cloves

1 cup washed kasha

1 tblsp. salt

12 teaspoon black pepper, freshly ground

3 cups veggie broth or water

4 cups chopped kale, stemmed and well cleaned

1. Combine the olive oil, squash, fennel, leeks, garlic, kasha, salt, pepper, and water in a slow cooker. Set the timer for 4 hours on high.

2. Add the kale just before serving. The stew's heat will cause it to wilt, making it easier to chew and digest.

PALEO TIP: Omit the kasha and use chicken broth instead of water or vegetable broth. Combine the other ingredients in a slow cooker with 1 pound mild Italian turkey sausage sliced into 1-inch pieces.

ACTION PLAN TIP: If you're following the Vegan, Mediterranean, or Time-Saving Action Plans, double the recipe to ensure you have enough leftovers for the rest of the week.

EACH SERVING

325 calories; 6 grammes of total fat

60g total carbohydrates

2 g sugar; 8 g fibre

12g protein; 1231mg sodium

Chapter Twenty-four

Beans with Chicken Chili

6 SERVINGS / 15 MINUTES TO PREPARE / 4 HOURS TO COOK

• THE MEDIEVAL

• SAVING TIME

Chicken chilli is a family favourite, and when served over brown rice or cooked quinoa, it can be extremely filling. The modest amount of chipotle powder adds a subtle spiciness to the dish, but not too much for those who prefer their meal mild. This recipe easily doubles (or triples!). For a quick supper or to take to work for lunches, freeze additional portions in single-serving containers.

2 tbsp olive oil extra-virgin

2 chopped onions

4 minced garlic cloves

2 chopped celery stalks

2 tablespoons cumin powder

1 tblsp. salt

1 teaspoon powdered chipotle

12 teaspoon black pepper, freshly ground

4 chicken breasts, boneless and skinless, cut into 1-inch pieces

1 teaspoon oregano, dry

1 leaf of bay

1 chopped tomato (28-ounce can)

2 12 cup chicken broth (plus more as needed)

2 (15-ounce) cans drained and rinsed white beans

14 cup fresh chopped parsley, divided

1. Toss the olive oil, onions, garlic, celery, cumin, salt, chipotle powder, pepper, chicken, oregano, bay leaf, tomatoes, chicken broth, and white beans together in a slow cooker. Preheat the oven to high and cook for 4 hours.

2. Add a bit more chicken broth or water if the mixture becomes too thick.

3. Sprinkle parsley on top of each serving. Serve on its own or with brown rice or quinoa.

Alert for Sensitivity

If you're following the Vegan Action Plan, leave out the chicken and replace it with vegetable broth instead.

EACH SERVING

423 calories; 13 grammes of total fat

Carbohydrates in total: 41g

6 g sugar; 10 g fibre

42g protein; 857mg sodium

Chapter Twenty-five

Stew with Mango and Black Beans

PREP TIME: 10 MINUTES / COOK TIME: 10 MINUTES / SERVES 4

• VEGETARIAN

• THE MEDIEVAL

Mangos alkalize your body and contain digestive enzymes. This stew is quick and easy to make, and it tastes great. Leftovers can be used as a topping for grilled poultry or seafood, as well as eaten alone.

coconut oil, 2 tablespoons

1 chopped onion

2 (15-ounce) cans drained and rinsed black beans

1 tablespoon cayenne pepper

1 tblsp. salt

14 teaspoon black pepper, freshly ground

1 cup of liquid

2 ripe mangos, thinly sliced

14 cup cilantro, chopped, divided

14 cup scallions, cut, divided

1. Melt the coconut oil in a big pot over high heat.

2. Cook for 5 minutes after adding the onion.

3. Combine the black beans, chilli powder, salt, pepper, and water in a large mixing bowl. Bring the water to a boil. Reduce the heat to low and continue to cook for another 5 minutes.

4. Remove the pot from the heat and, shortly before serving, mix in the mangos. Serve with cilantro and scallions on the side.

ACTION PLAN TIP: If you're following the Vegan Action Plan, double the recipe to ensure you have enough leftovers for the rest of the week.

EACH SERVING

431 calories; 9 grammes of total fat

72g total carbohydrates

17g sugar; 22g fibre

20g protein; 609mg sodium

Chapter Twenty-six

Stew with Coconut Fish

PREP TIME: 15 MINUTES / COOK TIME: 10 MINUTES / SERVES 4

- PALEO Diet
- THE MEDIEVAL

This dish gives your Action Plan a unique flavour. Many Pacific Rim cuisines include lemongrass. It is said to help digestion and decrease blood pressure. It has a delicate lemony flavour that complements the other flavours in the dish. While cooking in the broth, it is bruised to release its essential oils. Before serving, remember to remove the stalk.

coconut oil, 2 tablespoons

1 thinly sliced white onion

2 thinly chopped garlic cloves

2 thinly sliced zucchini

12 pound fillet of firm white fish, cut into 1-inch cubes

1 (4-inch) piece lemongrass, bruised with the back of a knife (white part only)

1 coconut milk can (13.5 oz.)

1 tblsp. salt

14 teaspoon white pepper, freshly ground

12 cup scallions, sliced

14 cup cilantro, chopped

3 tbsp lemon juice, freshly squeezed

1. Melt the coconut oil in a large pot over medium heat.

2. Add the zucchini, onion, and garlic. 5 minutes of sautéing

3. In a large pot, combine the fish, lemongrass, coconut milk, salt, and white pepper. If the liquid isn't enough to cover the fish, add more water. Bring to a boil, then reduce to a low heat and continue cooking for 5 minutes.

4. Add the scallions, cilantro, and lemon juice to the soup as garnish.

COOKING TIP: Add 1 teaspoon red pepper flakes if you prefer it spicy.

Replace the beans with 2 cups each cubed zucchini and cauliflower if you're following the Paleo Action Plan.

TIP: If you're following the Mediterranean or Time-Saving Action Plans, double the recipe to ensure you have enough leftovers for the rest of the week.

EACH SERVING

608 calories; 43 grammes of total fat

13g total carbohydrates

7g sugar; 4g fibre

46g protein; 725mg sodium

Chapter Twenty-seven

Salad with sliced apples, beets, and celery

PREP TIME: 15 MINUTES / SERVES 4

- VEGETARIAN
- PALEO Diet
- THE MEDIEVAL
- SAVING TIME

You haven't tasted this salad if you think you don't like beets. The remaining ingredients will most likely turn the same colour as the beets if there are any leftovers. There's no need to be concerned; you may still eat it. The ideal method to slice the vegetables is using a mandoline, but a food processor's slicing disc would suffice.

2 cored and quartered green apples

2 peeled and quartered tiny beets

four cups of spinach

2 thinly sliced celery stalks

12 red onion, thinly sliced

12 cup carrots, shredded

apple cider vinegar, 1 tbsp

1 tablespoon maple syrup or raw honey

extra-virgin olive oil, 3 teaspoons

Salt

black pepper, freshly ground

a quarter cup of pumpkin seeds

1. Slice the apples and beets using a mandoline or the slicing disc of a food processor.

2. Spread the spinach out on a big serving plate. Over the spinach, arrange the apples and beets. Add the celery, red onion, and carrots on top.

3. Whisk together the cider vinegar, honey, and olive oil in a small bowl. Salt & pepper to taste.

4. Toss the salad with the dressing and top with the pumpkin seeds.

If you're following the Vegan Action Plan, you can substitute maple syrup for honey.

ACTION PLAN TIP: If you're following the Vegan, Paleo, or Time-Saving Action Plans, double the recipe to ensure you have enough leftovers for the rest of the week.

EACH SERVING

239 calories; 15 grammes of total fat

27g total carbohydrates

18g sugar; 5g fibre

4g protein; 121mg sodium

Chapter Twenty-eight

Salad with Avocado and Mango

PREP TIME: 15 MINUTES / SERVES 4

- VEGETARIAN
- PALEO Diet
- THE MEDIEVAL
- SAVING TIME

This salad is light and refreshing, with plenty of healthful fats and fibre. Garnish with toasted slivered almonds and shredded coconut for added crunch. This is a wonderful breakfast salad if you want to experiment with different ingredients in the morning.

2 chopped romaine lettuce hearts

1 peeled cucumber, cut into 14-inch chunks

2 ripe mangos, sliced

12 in. cubes

2 thinly sliced scallions

1 avocado, large and ripe

1 cup dressing (creamy coconut-herb) (see here)

1. Toss the romaine lettuce, cucumber, mangos, onions, and avocado in a large serving bowl.

2. Toss the fruit and vegetables with the Creamy Coconut-Herb Dressing. Toss everything together.

PALEO & MEDITERRANEAN TIP: Add grilled chicken or fish to make this an entrée salad for people following the Mediterranean and Paleo Action Plans.

EACH SERVING

253 calories; 13 grammes of total fat

37g total carbohydrates

21g sugar; 10g fibre

4g protein; 363mg sodium

Chapter Twenty-nine

Salad Almost Caesar

PREP TIME: 15 MINUTES / SERVES 4

- PALEO Diet
- THE MEDIEVAL
- SAVING TIME

A restaurant Caesar salad is unquestionably laden with croutons, eggs, and shaved Parmesan cheese. This recipe has all of the original Caesar flavours but none of the inflammatory items. The crunch of the sunflower seeds substitutes the croutons, and the hearts of palm give a wonderful tang.

2 chopped romaine lettuce hearts

1 (14-ounce) can drained and sliced hearts of palm

12 CUP SUNSHINE SEEDS

1 Almost Caesar Dressing recipe (see here)

Salt

black pepper, freshly ground

1. Toss the romaine lettuce, hearts of palm, and sunflower seeds together in a large mixing basin.

2. Drizzle just enough dressing over the lettuce leaves to lightly cover them. Save any leftover dressing for another occasion.

3. Season with salt and pepper before serving.

If you're following the Vegan Action Plan, you may make the Almost Caesar Dressing with olives instead of anchovies (see here).

PALEO & MEDITERRANEAN TIP: Add grilled chicken to make this an entrée salad for those following the Mediterranean and Paleo Action Plans.

EACH SERVING

431 calories; 42 grammes of total fat

14g total carbohydrates

3 g sugar; 5 g fibre

6g protein; 803mg sodium

Chapter Thirty

Slaw of Brussels Sprouts

PREP TIME: 15 MINUTES / SERVES 4

- VEGETARIAN
- PALEO Diet
- THE MEDIEVAL
- SAVING TIME

Many individuals grew up despising those apparently "healthy" Brussels sprouts that were frequently overdone. This is how you eat them if you're one of those folks. This crisp slaw is a great accompaniment to roasted chicken or turkey. If pomegranate seeds aren't available, dried cherries can be used instead.

1 pound Brussels sprouts, stems cut off and thinly sliced

12 red onion, thinly sliced

1 apple, cored and thinly sliced

1 teaspoon mustard (Dijon)

1 tblsp. salt

1 tablespoon maple syrup or raw honey

apple cider vinegar, 2 tablespoons

1 cup yoghurt made with coconut milk

12 cup toasted hazelnuts, chopped

pomegranate seeds (12 cup)

1. Combine the Brussels sprouts, onion, and apple in a medium mixing basin.

2. Combine the Dijon mustard, salt, honey, cider vinegar, and yoghurt in a small bowl.

3. Toss the Brussels sprouts with the dressing until they are equally covered.

4. Sprinkle the hazelnuts and pomegranate seeds on top of the salad.

Alert for Sensitivity

COOKING TIP: Let this slaw sit for 30 minutes before serving to increase the flavour.

If you're following the Vegan Action Plan, you can substitute maple syrup for honey.

EACH SERVING

189 calories; 8 grammes of total fat

29g total carbohydrates

13 g sugar; 9 g fibre

6g protein; 678mg sodium

Chapter Thirty-one

Feta Cheese and Vegetable Slaw

4–6 SERVINGS / PREP TIME: 20 MINUTES

• VEGETARIAN

• THE MEDIEVAL

This slaw is a delicious way to get your veggies. This colourful and antioxidant-rich salad contains shredded broccoli, carrots, celery root, beets, zucchini, and red onions. The prep is made easier using a food processor shredding disc. Use any vegetables you choose in this slaw.

12 cup olive oil (extra virgin)

12 gallon apple cider vinegar

1 tablespoon maple syrup or raw honey

1 teaspoon mustard (Dijon)

1 tblsp. salt

14 teaspoon black pepper, freshly ground

2 big peeled and chopped broccoli stems

2 peeled and shredded carrots

12 peeled and chopped celery root bulb

1 big peeled and shredded beet

2 shredded zucchini

1 small red onion, thinly sliced

14 cup fresh Italian parsley, chopped

3 oz. crumbled feta cheese

1. Whisk together the olive oil, cider vinegar, honey, Dijon mustard, salt, and pepper in a large mixing basin.

2. Combine the broccoli, carrots, celery root, beets, zucchini, onion, and parsley in a large mixing bowl. Toss the vegetables in the dressing to coat them.

3. To serve, place the slaw in a serving bowl and top with feta cheese.

VEGAN & PALEO TIP: If you don't want to use feta cheese, use cashew cheese instead.

If you're following the Vegan Action Plan, you can substitute maple syrup for honey.

EACH SERVING

388 calories; 30 grammes of total fat

26g total carbohydrates

12 g sugar; 6 g fibre

8g protein; 981mg sodium

Chopped Mediterranean Salad

PREP TIME: 15 MINUTES / SERVES 4

- VEGETARIAN
- PALEO Diet
- THE MEDIEVAL
- SAVING TIME

This version is based on fattoush, a flatbread and vegetable salad, but without the flatbread. A traditional addition in this salad is sumac, a Middle Eastern spice. It has a citrus flavour to it. The salad is light and delicious, and it goes well with lamb. Add drained garbanzo beans or white beans for more protein.

2 cups spinach, packed

3 big sliced tomatoes

1 bunch thinly sliced radishes

1 peeled and diced English cucumber

2 sliced scallions

2 minced garlic cloves

1 tablespoon fresh mint, chopped

1 tablespoon parsley, chopped

1 cup plain unsweetened almond yoghurt

¼ cup extra-virgin olive oil

3 tbsp lemon juice, freshly squeezed

apple cider vinegar, 1 tbsp

1 tblsp. salt

14 teaspoon black pepper, freshly ground

1 teaspoon of sumac

Toss the spinach, tomatoes, radishes, cucumber, scallions, garlic, mint, parsley, yoghurt, olive oil, lemon juice, cider vinegar, salt, and sumac together in a large mixing basin. Toss everything together.

PALEO & MEDITERRANEAN TIP: Add cooked chicken or fish to make this an entrée salad for the Mediterranean or Paleo Action Plans.

MEDITERRANEAN TIP: Crumble 3 ounces of goat cheese on top if following the Mediterranean Action Plan.

ACTION PLAN TIP: If you're following the Vegan, Paleo, Mediterranean, or Time-Saving Action Plans, double the recipe to ensure you have enough leftovers for the rest of the week.

EACH SERVING

194 calories; 14 grammes of total fat

15g total carbohydrates

7 g sugar; 5 g fibre

4g protein; 661mg sodium

Chapter Thirty-two

Salad with Quinoa and Roasted Asparagus

PREP TIME: 10 MINUTES / COOK TIME: 15 MINUTES / SERVES 4

• VEGETARIAN

• THE MEDIEVAL

This dish will quickly become a favourite. Use precooked quinoa, which can be found in the frozen food section of most supermarkets. The asparagus flavour is enhanced by roasting it, and the flaxseed adds crunch and nuttiness to the salad.

1 asparagus bunch, trimmed

3 tbsp extra-virgin olive oil (divided)

1 teaspoon salt, plus more as needed for seasoning

2 cups cold or room temperature cooked quinoa

14 finely chopped red onion

apple cider vinegar, 1 tbsp

14 cup fresh mint, chopped

flaxseed, 1 tbsp

black pepper, freshly ground

1. Preheat the oven to 400 degrees Fahrenheit.

2. Toss the asparagus with 1 tablespoon olive oil and 1 teaspoon salt in a large mixing basin.

3. Wrap the asparagus in a single layer of aluminium foil and place it on a baking pan. Roast the asparagus for 10 to 15 minutes on a baking sheet in a preheated oven.

4. In a large mixing bowl, combine the quinoa, onion, vinegar, mint, flaxseed, and the remaining 2 tablespoons of olive oil while the asparagus is roasting.

5. Slice the asparagus into 12-inch sections once it has cooled enough to handle. Season with salt and pepper before adding to the quinoa.

EACH SERVING

228 calories; 13 g total fat

24g total carbohydrates

2 g sugar; 5 g fibre

6g protein; 592mg sodium

Chapter Thirty-three

Salad with White Beans and Tuna

PREP TIME: 15 MINUTES / SERVES 4

• THE MEDIEVAL

• SAVING TIME

This is a "pantry salad," because all of the components are likely to be found in your well-stocked pantry. If you cook this salad ahead of time, the flavours will intensify. If cooking ahead, wait until just before serving to add the tomatoes and arugula.

arugula, 4 cups

2 cans (5 oz.) flaked white tuna, drained

1 can (15 oz.) white beans, rinsed and drained

12 pint cherry tomatoes, lengthwise halved

12 finely sliced red onion

12 cup Kalamata olives, pitted

14 cup olive oil (extra virgin)

2 tbsp lemon juice, freshly squeezed

Salt

black pepper, freshly ground

2 oz. crumbled feta cheese (from sheep's milk or goat's milk)

1. Combine the arugula, tuna, white beans, tomatoes, onion, olives, olive oil, and lemon juice in a large mixing basin. Salt & pepper to taste.

2. Top the salad with feta cheese just before serving.

PALEO TIP: Remove the white beans and feta cheese from the recipe.

ACTION PLAN TIP: If you're using this recipe as part of the Time-Saving Action Plan, double the quantities to ensure you have leftovers for the rest of the week.

EACH SERVING

373 calories; 19g total fat

28g total carbohydrates

3 g sugar; 7 g fibre

29g protein; 388mg sodium

Chapter Thirty-four

Salsa de Mango

PREP TIME: 15 MINUTES / MAKES ABOUT 2 CUPS

• VEGETARIAN

• PALEO Diet

• THE MEDIEVAL

• SAVING TIME

Almost any dish—or party—will benefit from this salsa. Fish, chicken, tacos, and salads all benefit from it. Mangos are high in vitamins A and C, as well as probiotic fibre. Make this with papaya instead of mangos or a combination of the two.

2 cups mango chunks

12 cup red onion, minced

14 cup fresh cilantro, chopped

1 minced garlic clove

1 tablespoon lemon juice, freshly squeezed

1 tsp salt

1. Combine the mango, onion, cilantro, garlic, lemon juice, and salt in a medium mixing basin.

2. Refrigerate for up to one week in an airtight container.

14 CUP PER SERVING

40 calories; 0 grammes of total fat

10g total carbohydrates

8 g sugar; 1 g fibre

Sodium: 98mg; Protein: 0g

Chapter Thirty-five

Root Vegetables Roasted

PREP TIME: 15 MINUTES / COOK TIME: 25 TO 35 MINUTES / SERVES 4 TO 6

• VEGETARIAN

• PALEO Diet

• THE MEDIEVAL

Even the pickiest diners will accept root veggies when they are roasted. The vegetables grow sweeter and richer in flavour, while the outsides become slightly crispy, brown, and delectable. Roasted Vegetable Soup can be made using any leftovers (see here).

2 small sweet potatoes, peeled and sliced into 1-inch chunks

1 bunch peeled and cut into 1-inch cubes of beets

4 peeled carrots, cut into 1-inch rounds

3 peeled parsnips, sliced into 1-inch rounds

14 cup melted coconut oil

1 tablespoon olive oil (extra virgin)

1 tablespoon maple syrup or raw honey

1 tblsp. salt

12 teaspoon black pepper, freshly ground

1. Preheat the oven to 400 degrees Fahrenheit.

2. Use parchment paper to line two rimmed baking sheets.

3. Combine the sweet potatoes, beets, carrots, and parsnips in a large mixing bowl. Combine the coconut oil, olive oil, honey, salt, and pepper in a mixing bowl. Toss the vegetables to coat them.

4. Distribute the vegetables evenly between the two baking sheets, forming a single layer.

5. Bake the vegetables for 10 to 15 minutes on the sheets in a preheated oven. Turn them over so the other side browns. Bake for another 10 to 15 minutes, or until the vegetables are golden and soft. Warm or at room temperature is fine.

COOKING TIP: Remove the vegetables from the oven if they are brown but not fully done. Allow the vegetables to steam for about 10 minutes after covering them with aluminium foil.

In addition, the fresher the vegetables are, the less time they will take to roast.

If you're following the Vegan Action Plan, you can substitute maple syrup for honey.

EACH SERVING

460 calories; 18 grammes of total fat

74g total carbohydrates

23g sugar; 14g fibre

6g protein; 760mg sodium

Chapter Thirty-six

Salad with Turmeric Chicken

PREP TIME: 15 MINUTES / COOK TIME: 20 MINUTES / SERVES 4

- PALEO Diet
- THE MEDIEVAL
- SAVING TIME

Turmeric, which is used in the spice rub for the chicken, has anti-inflammatory properties. This rub is also wonderful on salmon, which you could use in place of the chicken. For the finest flavour, marinate it for at least 30 minutes or overnight.

4 chicken breasts, boneless and skinless

1 tablespoon olive oil (extra virgin)

1 tablespoon cilantro, chopped

1 minced garlic clove

1 tblsp. salt

14 teaspoon turmeric powder

14 teaspoon black pepper, freshly ground

12 cup almond yoghurt, unsweetened

1 tablespoon lemon juice, freshly squeezed

1 teaspoon zest of lemon

12 cup almonds, chopped

6 cups romaine lettuce, chopped

1. Place the chicken breasts in a small baking dish.

2. Whisk together the olive oil, cilantro, garlic, salt, turmeric, and pepper in a small bowl. Rub the chicken with the mixture. Cover the chicken and marinate for at least 30 minutes or overnight in the refrigerator.

3. Preheat the oven to 375 degrees Fahrenheit. Place the baking dish in the preheated oven and bake the chicken for 20 minutes once the oven is hot. Take it out of the oven and set it aside.

4. Whisk together the yoghurt, lemon juice, and lemon zest in a large mixing bowl. Toss in the almonds and romaine lettuce to evenly distribute the dressing.

5. Place the salad on a serving plate and serve. Cut the chicken breasts into strips and place them on top of the lettuce.

Alert for Sensitivity

TIME SAVING TIP: Cook the chicken ahead of time and serve it cold over the salad.

Instead of chicken, toss a can of drained garbanzo or white beans with the olive oil, cilantro, garlic, salt, turmeric, and pepper and serve over the yogurt-dressed greens.

EACH SERVING

418 calories; 21 grammes of total fat

10g total carbohydrates

3 g sugar; 4 g fibre

46g protein; 759mg sodium

Chapter Thirty-seven

Bowl of lentils, vegetables, and fruit

4–6 SERVINGS / PREP TIME: 20 MINUTES

• VEGETARIAN

• THE MEDIEVAL

A unique take on the traditional brown rice and lentil dish. Red lentils that have been soaked overnight are paired with jicama and pear in this dish. This salad's base can be prepared the night before, and the fruits and veggies can be added the next day.

1 cup lentils (red)

2 quarts of water

4 cups brown rice, cooked

1 (15-ounce) can drained and washed lentils

sauce for chicken lettuce wraps (see here)

1 radish head, cored and ripped into pieces, divided

1 small jicama, peeled and divided into thin sticks

2 ripe red Bartlett (or other) pears, cored, quartered, and sliced

2 cut and split scallions

1. Combine the red lentils and water in a medium mixing dish. Refrigerate overnight, covered. When you're ready to make the salad, drain the lentils.

2. Combine the brown rice and canned lentils in a medium mixing bowl. Half of the Chicken Lettuce Wraps sauce should be added now. Allow for at least 30 minutes of rest time, or overnight.

3. In serving bowls, divide the lentil-rice mixture. Add equal portions of soaked and drained red lentils to each bowl. Serve with radicchio, jicama, pears, and scallions on the side.

4. Drizzle some of the remaining Chicken Lettuce Wraps sauce over each one.

EACH SERVING

989 calories; 31 grammes of total fat

151g total carbohydrates

16 g sugar; 35 g fibre

31g protein; 272mg sodium

Chapter Thirty-eight

Cauliflower with Almond Sauce, Roasted

PREP TIME: 15 MINUTES / COOK TIME: 20 MINUTES / SERVES 4

• VEGETARIAN

• PALEO Diet

• THE MEDIEVAL

Cauliflower is soft on the inside and crunchy on the outside after roasting. It's even better with almond sauce. This can be served warm or cold, as a salad or a side dish.

1 cauliflower head (cut into florets)

14 cup olive oil (extra virgin)

12 teaspoon turmeric powder

12 tablespoons salt (distributed)

12 teaspoon black pepper, freshly ground, divided

1 cup almond yoghurt, unsweetened

a quarter cup of almond butter

1 chopped scallion

1 minced garlic clove

1 tablespoon parsley, chopped

1 tablespoon lemon juice, freshly squeezed

1 teaspoon maple sugar

1. Preheat the oven to 400 degrees Fahrenheit.

2. Combine the cauliflower, olive oil, turmeric, 1 teaspoon salt, and 14 teaspoon pepper in a large mixing basin.

3. Arrange the seasoned cauliflower in a single layer on a rimmed baking sheet. Roast for 20 to 30 minutes, or until the cauliflower is lightly browned and soft, on a baking sheet in a preheated oven.

4. Combine the yoghurt, almond butter, scallions, garlic, parsley, lemon juice, maple syrup, the remaining 12 teaspoon salt, and the remaining 14 teaspoon pepper in a blender and mix until smooth. Purée until completely smooth.

5. Spread the almond sauce over the roasted cauliflower in a serving dish.

COOKING TIP: Use pomegranate seeds as a garnish when they're in season.

EACH SERVING

277 calories; 23 grammes of total fat

15g total carbohydrates

6 g sugar; 4 g fibre

7g protein; 945mg sodium

Purée de Cauliflower

PREP TIME: 15 MINUTES / COOK TIME: 10 MINUTES / SERVES 4

- VEGETARIAN
- PALEO Diet
- THE MEDIEVAL

Cauliflower purée is a delicious alternative to mashed potatoes and pairs well with grilled fish and meat. This dish goes well with roasted veggies and can also be used to make a vegan soup. Make a double batch and keep the extras in the freezer for a quick dinner addition.

1 cauliflower head, cut into florets

1 clove garlic

2 tablespoons salt (distributed)

14 teaspoon black pepper, freshly ground

12 gallon coconut milk

1 tablespoon olive oil (extra virgin)

1. Over high heat, bring a large saucepan of water to a boil. 1 teaspoon salt, the cauliflower, and the garlic clove Cook for 5 minutes, or until the cauliflower is soft.

2. Drain the cauliflower and garlic clove into a large mixing dish. Using a potato masher, mash the potatoes.

3. Toss the mash with the remaining 1 teaspoon of salt, the pepper, and the coconut milk. Stir until everything is completely blended.

4. Drizzle some olive oil over the purée in a serving bowl.

COOKING TIP: In a food processor, puree the cooked cauliflower, garlic, salt, pepper, and coconut milk until smooth.

EACH SERVING

117 calories; 11 grammes of total fat

6 g total carbohydrates

3 g sugar; 2 g fibre

2g protein; 1187mg sodium

Chapter Thirty-nine

Crispy Shallots with Green Beans

PREP TIME: 10 MINUTES / COOK TIME: 15 MINUTES / SERVES 4

• VEGETARIAN

• PALEO Diet

• THE MEDIEVAL

As the shallots crisp in the oil, they impart a wonderful, delicate allium taste to the beans. This recipe is a great complement to any entrée and will elevate your dinner experience.

1 teaspoon sea salt, plus more as needed for seasoning

1 pound trimmed green beans

14 cup olive oil (extra virgin)

1 shallot, thinly sliced

1 tablespoon tarragon, chopped

black pepper, freshly ground

1. Over high heat, bring a large saucepan of water to a boil.

2. Toss the beans into the boiling water with 1 teaspoon of sea salt. Cook for approximately 5 minutes, or until bright green.

3. Drain and transfer the beans to a serving dish.

4. Heat the olive oil in a small saucepan over medium heat. Add the shallots after the oil is heated. Cook for 1 to 2 minutes, or until browning begins.

5. Over the green beans, scatter the shallots. Season with sea salt and pepper after adding the tarragon.

EACH SERVING

146 calories; 13 grammes of total fat

9g total carbohydrates

2 g sugar; 4 g fibre

2g protein; 475mg sodium

Chapter Forty

Pineapple and Roasted Sweet Potatoes

PREP TIME: 15 MINUTES / COOK TIME: 25 MINUTES / SERVES 4

• VEGETARIAN

• PALEO Diet

• THE MEDIEVAL

This recipe represents yin and yang in the kitchen. The sweet potatoes are seasoned with curry powder, and roasting them with pineapple brings out the curry powder's greatest tastes. Pineapple is a sweet, juicy fruit that is high in vitamin C and improves digestion. This is a light supper on its alone, but it also goes well with chicken, salmon, or swordfish.

coconut oil, 3 teaspoons

2 large peeled and cut into 12-inch chunks sweet potatoes or yams

1 cup pineapple, cut into 12 inch chunks

curry powder (two teaspoons)

1 tblsp. salt

14 teaspoon black pepper, freshly ground

1. Preheat the oven to 400 degrees Fahrenheit.

2. Microwave the coconut oil for about 1 minute on high in a microwave-safe bowl.

3. Combine the sweet potatoes and pineapple in a large mixing dish. Add the curry powder, salt, and pepper to the melted coconut oil. Toss everything together.

4. Fill a rimmed baking sheet halfway with the mixture. Roast for 20 to 25 minutes, or until the sweet potatoes are soft, on a baking sheet in a preheated oven.

5. Warm or at room temperature is fine.

TIP: Use pre-cut sweet potatoes and pineapple from the produce section of most supermarkets to save time.

ACTION PLAN TIP: If you're following the Vegan Action Plan, double the recipe to ensure you have enough leftovers for the rest of the week.

EACH SERVING

230 calories; 11 grammes of total fat

34g total carbohydrates

5 g sugar; 5 g fibre

2g protein; 591mg sodium

Chapter Forty-one

Sauté Quinoa-Broccolini

PREP TIME: 10 MINUTES / COOK TIME: 10 MINUTES / SERVES 4

• VEGETARIAN

• THE MEDIEVAL

This recipe is quick and easy to prepare. Broccolini, often known as baby broccoli, is a versatile vegetable with smaller, more sensitive stalks than typical broccoli, resulting in less waste. This dinner comes together quickly thanks to the precooked quinoa, and you can add cooked lentils for added protein.

coconut oil, 1 tablespoon

2 leeks, cut white portion only

2 chopped garlic cloves

4 cups broccolini, chopped

12 cup water or vegetable broth

curry powder (1 teaspoon)

2 cups quinoa, cooked

1 tablespoon amino acids de coco

1. Melt the coconut oil in a large skillet over high heat. Add the garlic and leeks. 2 minutes of sautéing

2. Combine the broccolini with the vegetable broth. Cook for 5 minutes with the lid on.

3. Combine the curry powder, quinoa, and coconut aminos in a mixing bowl. Cook, uncovered, for 2 to 3 minutes, or until the quinoa is warmed through.

4. Serve as a salad at room temperature or warm as a side dish.

EACH SERVING

273 calories; 6 grammes of total fat

44g total carbohydrates

5 g sugar; 6 g fibre

11g protein; 54mg sodium

Chapter Forty-two

Bok Choy Braised with Shiitake Mushrooms

PREP TIME: 10 MINUTES / COOK TIME: 10 MINUTES / SERVES 4

- VEGETARIAN
- PALEO Diet
- THE MEDIEVAL

Consider ordering some not-so-healthy takeout. Instead, try this dish. Coconut aminos come from the sap or juice of a tapped coconut tree. It stands in for soy sauce here, bringing depth of flavour and a hint of sweetness.

coconut oil, 1 tablespoon

8 baby bok choy, lengthwise half

12 cup of water

1 tablespoon amino acids de coco

1 cup thinly sliced shiitake mushrooms, stemmed

Salt

black pepper, freshly ground

1 scallion, thinly sliced

1 tablespoon sesame seeds, roasted

1. Melt the coconut oil in a big pan over high heat. In a single layer, place the bok choy.

2. Fill the pan with water, coconut aminos, and mushrooms. Cover the vegetables and cook for 5 to 10 minutes, or until the bok choy is soft.

3. Take the pan off the heat. Add salt and pepper to the vegetables.

4. Place the bok choy and mushrooms on a serving platter and top with the scallions and sesame seeds.

PALEO & MEDITERRANEAN TIP: Instead of water, use chicken broth for individuals following the Mediterranean and Paleo Action Plans. If shiitake mushrooms aren't accessible or don't fit into your budget, you can substitute any other mushroom.

EACH SERVING

285 calories; 8 g total fat

43g total carbohydrates

21g sugar; 18g fibre

26g protein; 1185mg sodium

Chapter Forty-three

Broccoli and Cashews Roasted

PREP TIME: 10 MINUTES / COOK TIME: 20 MINUTES / SERVES 4

• VEGETARIAN

• PALEO Diet

• THE MEDIEVAL

Broccoli becomes somewhat crunchier and sweeter when roasted. The nuttiness comes from the coconut aminos and cashews. This meal is terrific at room temperature, making it a great potluck dish; it's also delicious when served warm.

broccoli florets, 6 cups

2 tbsp olive oil extra-virgin

1 tblsp. salt

1 tablespoon amino acids de coco

12 cup cashews, roasted

1. Preheat the oven to 375 degrees Fahrenheit.

2. Toss the broccoli with the olive oil and salt in a large mixing bowl. Place the broccoli on a baking pan and spread it out in a single layer. Roast for 15 to 20 minutes, or until the broccoli is cooked, on a baking sheet in a preheated oven.

3. Toss the roasted broccoli with the coconut aminos and cashews in a large mixing dish and serve.

Alert for Sensitivity

EACH SERVING

209 calories; 15 grammes of total fat

15g total carbohydrates

3 g sugar; 4 g fibre

6g protein; 633mg sodium

Chapter Forty-four

Hash with Ginger Sweet Potatoes and Peas

PREP TIME: 10 MINUTES / COOK TIME: 10 MINUTES / SERVES 4

• VEGETARIAN

• THE MEDIEVAL

Sweet potatoes and brown rice are seasoned with anti-inflammatory spices like ginger, curry, and turmeric in this hearty dish. This recipe saves time by using precooked sweet potatoes and cooked brown rice.

coconut oil, 2 tablespoons

4 sliced scallions

3 minced garlic cloves

2 teaspoons fresh ginger, minced

curry powder (1 teaspoon)

1 tblsp. salt

12 teaspoon turmeric powder

2 medium sweet potatoes, peeled and diced after roasting in their skins

1 cup peas, frozen

2 cups brown rice, cooked

1 tablespoon amino acids de coco

14 cup fresh cilantro, chopped

12 cup cashews, chopped

1. Melt the coconut oil in a large skillet over medium-high heat. Combine the scallions, garlic, ginger, curry powder, salt, and turmeric in a large mixing bowl. Cook for 2 minutes, or until aromatic.

2. Combine the sweet potatoes, peas, brown rice, and coconut aminos in a large mixing bowl. 5 minutes of sautéing

3. Place the hash on a serving platter and top with the cilantro and cashews.

Alert for Sensitivity

EACH SERVING

511 calories; 17 grammes of total fat

83g total carbohydrates

4 g sugar; 10 g fibre

11g protein; 633mg sodium

Chapter Forty-five

Bowl of Buddha

PREP TIME: 15 MINUTES / COOK TIME: 35 MINUTES / SERVES 4 TO 6

• VEGETARIAN

• THE MEDIEVAL

There are a few different versions of how this meal received its name. Some believe it's because it represents Buddha's full belly, while others claim it's because Zen monks walk door to door with a bowl receiving whatever food is offered. It's basically a dish of rice with whatever vegetables you choose and seasoned to your liking. It is simple and stress-free.

1 cup basmati brown rice

2 c. vegetable stock

3 tbsp coconut oil (distributed)

2 tablespoons salt (distributed)

1 pint mushrooms, sliced

2 thinly chopped garlic cloves

4 ounces stringless fresh snow peas

2 thinly sliced carrots

12 cup thawed frozen peas

2 thinly sliced scallions

3 tablespoons fresh cilantro, chopped

3 tablespoons lime juice, freshly squeezed

1 tablespoon sesame oil, roasted

1 tablespoon amino acids de coco

12 teaspoon crushed red pepper

1. In a medium saucepan over high heat, whisk together the basmati rice, vegetable broth, 1 tablespoon of coconut oil, and 1 teaspoon of salt. Bring to a boil, then turn down to a low heat. Cook the rice for 25 to 35 minutes, covered, or until soft.

2. Melt the remaining 2 tablespoons of coconut oil in a large pan over high heat. Toss in the mushrooms. Cook for 5 minutes, or until gently browned.

3. Garlic, snow peas, and carrots should be added now. Sauté for another 3 minutes. Cover the pan with the thawed peas to keep them heated.

4. Stir in the sautéed vegetables with the rice to mix. Add the scallions, cilantro, lime juice, sesame oil, coconut aminos, red pepper flakes, and the remaining 1 teaspoon of salt when ready to serve.

INGREDIENT TIP: Brown basmati rice is preferred in this dish since it cooks faster, but any type of brown rice will suffice. If you're worried about the rice boiling over, keep the lid slightly ajar as it cooks.

EACH SERVING

371 calories; 15 grammes of total fat

51g total carbohydrates

5 g sugar; 4 g fibre

9g protein; 1591mg sodium

Chapter Forty-six

Risotto with Mushrooms

PREP TIME: 15 MINUTES / COOK TIME: 20 MINUTES / SERVES 4

• VEGETARIAN

• THE MEDIEVAL

This recipe is for you if you enjoy Italian cuisine. Risotto has a reputation for being difficult to prepare, but this is not the case. The key is to slowly pour in the liquid while constantly stirring the rice. You'll have a warm, creamy, fulfilling supper once all of the liquid has been combined and the rice is tender. If arborio rice is unavailable, any short-grain white rice would suffice. Because of its tougher outer shell, brown rice is not suitable for risotto.

2 tbsp olive oil extra-virgin

1 big sliced shallot

1 minced garlic clove

1 pint mushrooms, sliced

12 cup rice arborio

3 cups warmed vegetable broth

1 tblsp. salt

12 teaspoon black pepper, freshly ground

a pinch of nutmeg

1 tablespoon thyme leaves, chopped

For garnish, balsamic vinegar

1. Heat the olive oil in a big skillet over high heat. Add the garlic and shallots. 3 minutes of sautéing

2. Add the rice and mushrooms. Sauté for another 3 minutes.

3. Reduce to medium-high heat. Add one cup of vegetable broth at a time, stirring continually until the liquid has been absorbed by the rice before adding another cup.

4. Add the salt, pepper, and nutmeg once all of the broth has been absorbed. Check the rice for doneness by tasting it; it should be soft but not mushy.

5. Place the risotto in a serving bowl. Drizzle with balsamic vinegar and garnish with thyme leaves.

COOKING TIP: If the rice isn't soft after using all of the broth, add more liquid (broth or water) a quarter cup at a time until it is. Cover the risotto, turn off the heat, and let it sit for 5 minutes if the rice is little underdone.

TIP: If you're following the Vegan or Mediterranean Action Plans, double the recipe to ensure you have enough leftovers for the rest of the week.

EACH SERVING

359 calories; 9 grammes of total fat

60g total carbohydrates

1 g sugar; 3 g fibre

10g protein; 1162mg sodium

CPSIA information can be obtained
at www.ICGtesting.com
Printed in the USA
LVHW061206190722
723853LV00014B/519

9 781804 769263